A Guide To Healing

Created to help you find inner peace.

"There is beauty that will
come of all things."
~Mary Neal

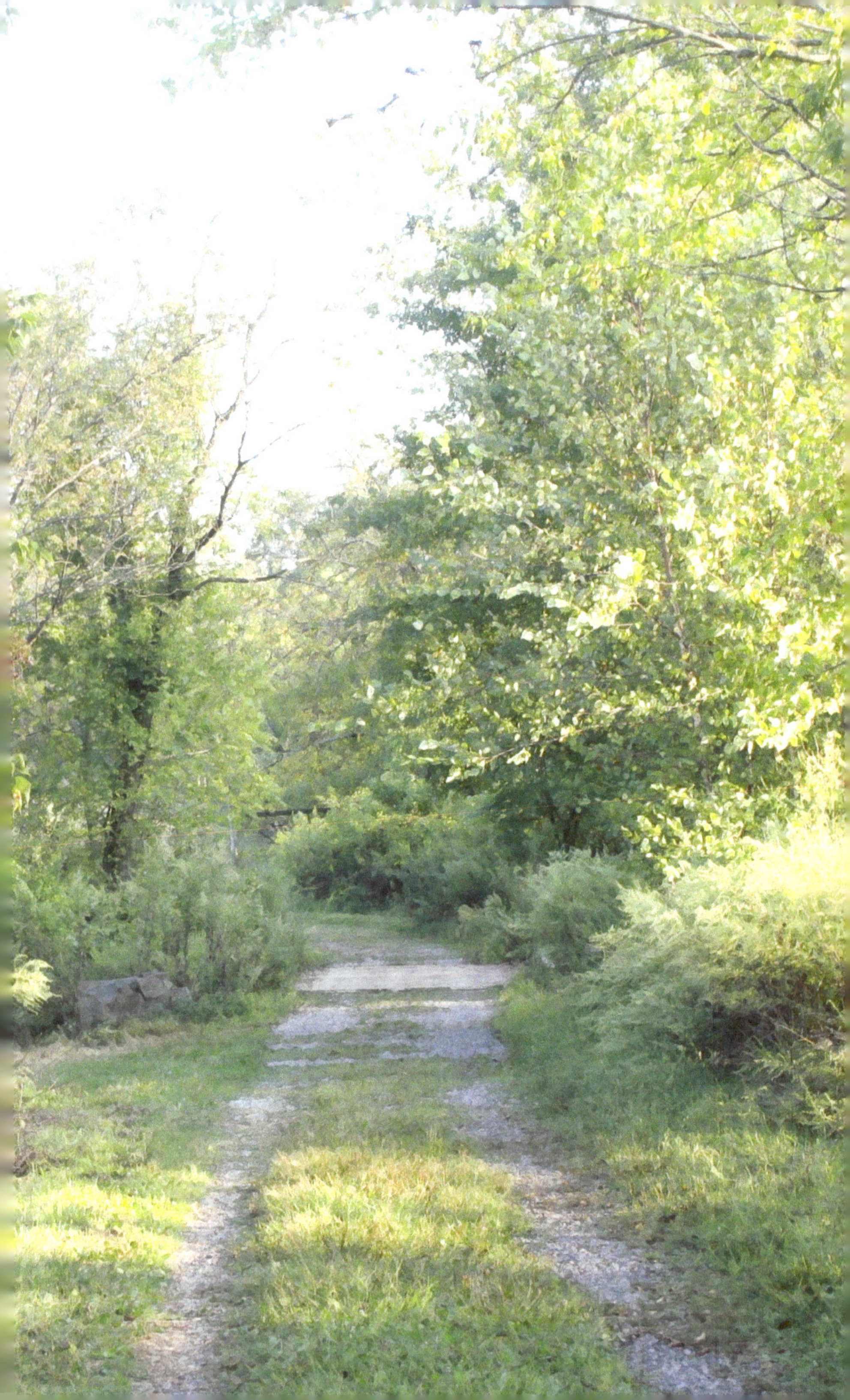

Table of Contents

Preface

When I told Celia, my good friend, health advocate and writer, about my idea to create a simple holistic healing guide that would support all types of people in all stages of healing, she agreed to help me make this vision a reality.

This guide was inspired by the many loved ones, clients and others I've watched struggle with declining health and lack of happiness, as well as my own personal journey. I KNOW firsthand that reaching a state of inner peace and well-being is not always easy. This is especially true if you are at war with your body, yourself or even your life.

I am passionate about helping people find inner peace and well-being. That's why I created this guide for YOU. It is based on my many years of training, experience, research and coaching. It also includes best practices from educators and experts in the holistic healing field. This guide will help you connect with knowledge, insight, understanding, gratitude, strength and Inner Peace as you embark on your own personal healing journey.

With So Much Peace and Love, Mary

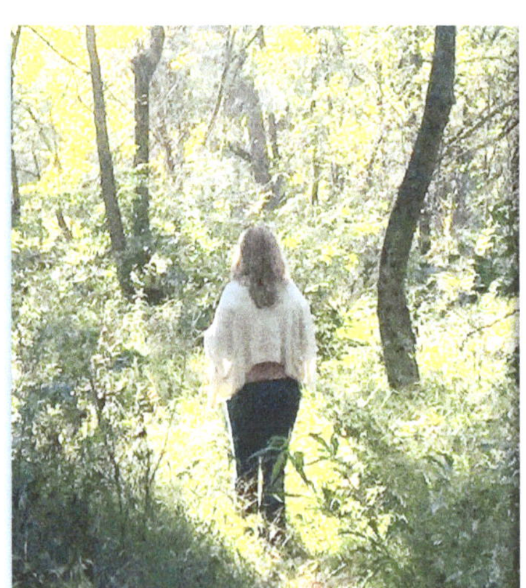

"Pursue some path, however narrow and crooked, in which you can walk with love and reverence."

~Henry David Thoreau

Introduction

Welcome to your healing journey, an adventure that is made up of **P**ausing, **E**xploring, **A**ligning, **C**hoosing and **E**xperiencing. In other words…a journey toward inner **P.E.A.C.E.**

I'm sorry if you're in a place of pain and/or struggle. No doubt sometimes life hurts. This pain is a part of life that we ALL go through at different crossroads, be it physical or emotional. I hold a very deep belief that our challenges offer the opportunity for personal growth and might even serve as a wake-up call. Then again, sometimes things just seem to happen.

Whatever the case, this simple guide is in your hands to help you on your journey and lead you to the path of inner PEACE, where you will find healing. Through beautiful images, nourishing affirmations, self-discovery and simple practices, you have the potential to become healthier, stronger, more balanced and peaceful...now, and for the rest of your life.

As with any journey, parts of the path may be smooth, easy and beautiful. Other parts may be rugged, rocky and even threatening. The key is to stick with it and go at your own pace keeping an open heart, an open mind, and compassion.

To get the most from this guide, you are encouraged to take one small step at a time. Be sure to track your progress while making sure you are being extra loving and patient toward yourself and others. Know that you have help and are surrounded by people who truly care.

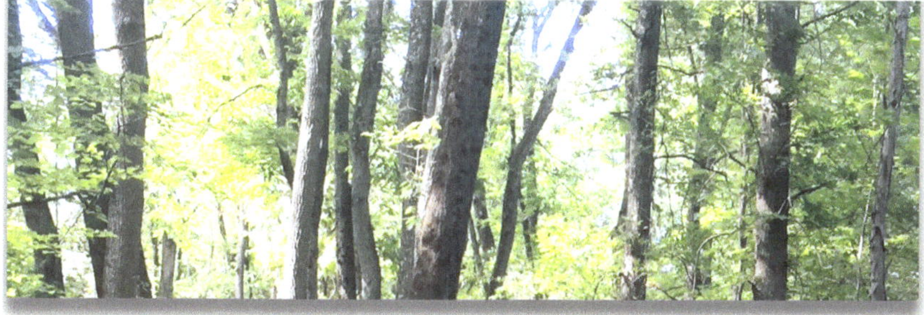

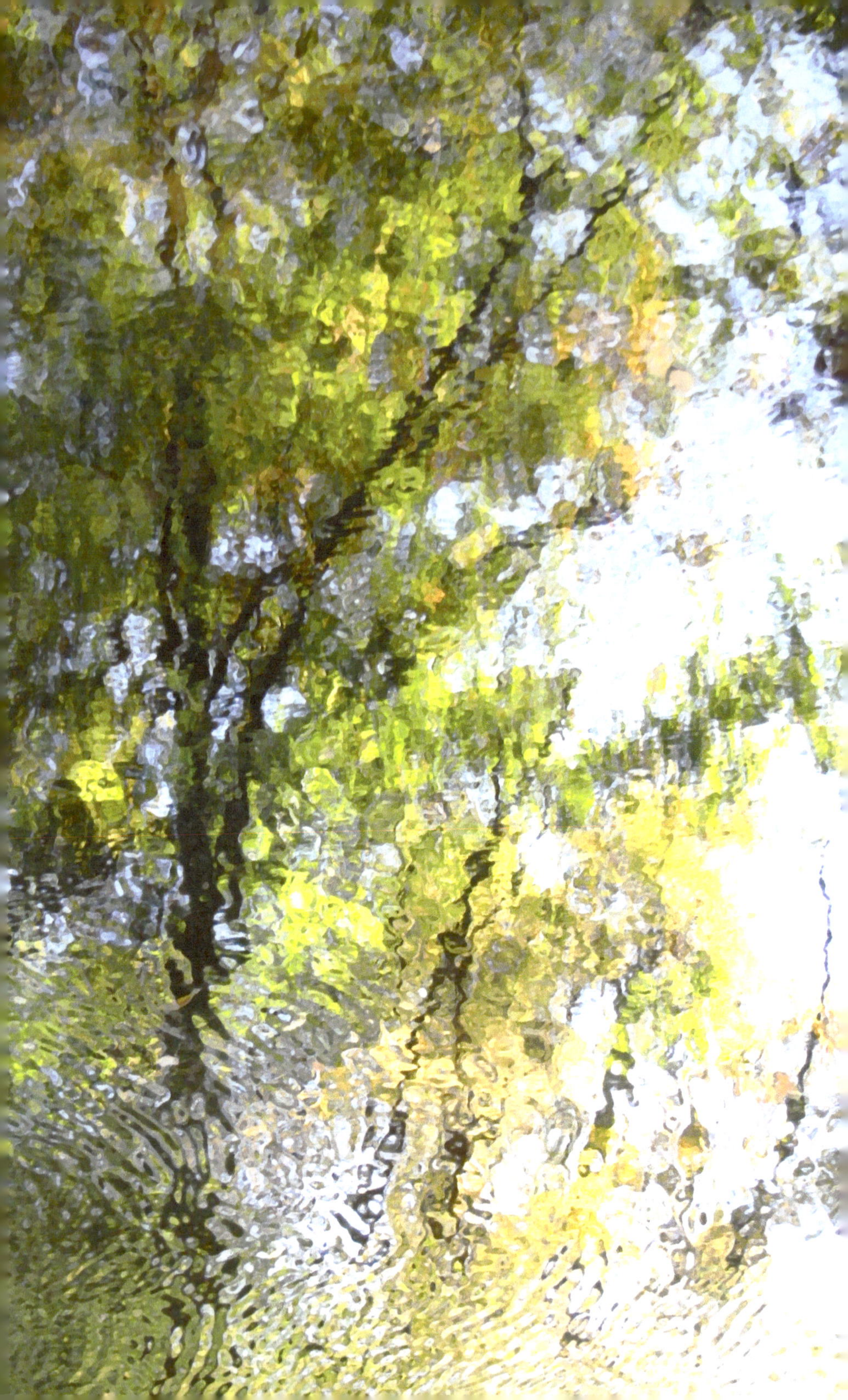

Your Time to PAUSE

"All that is important comes in
quietness and waiting."

~Patrick Lindsay

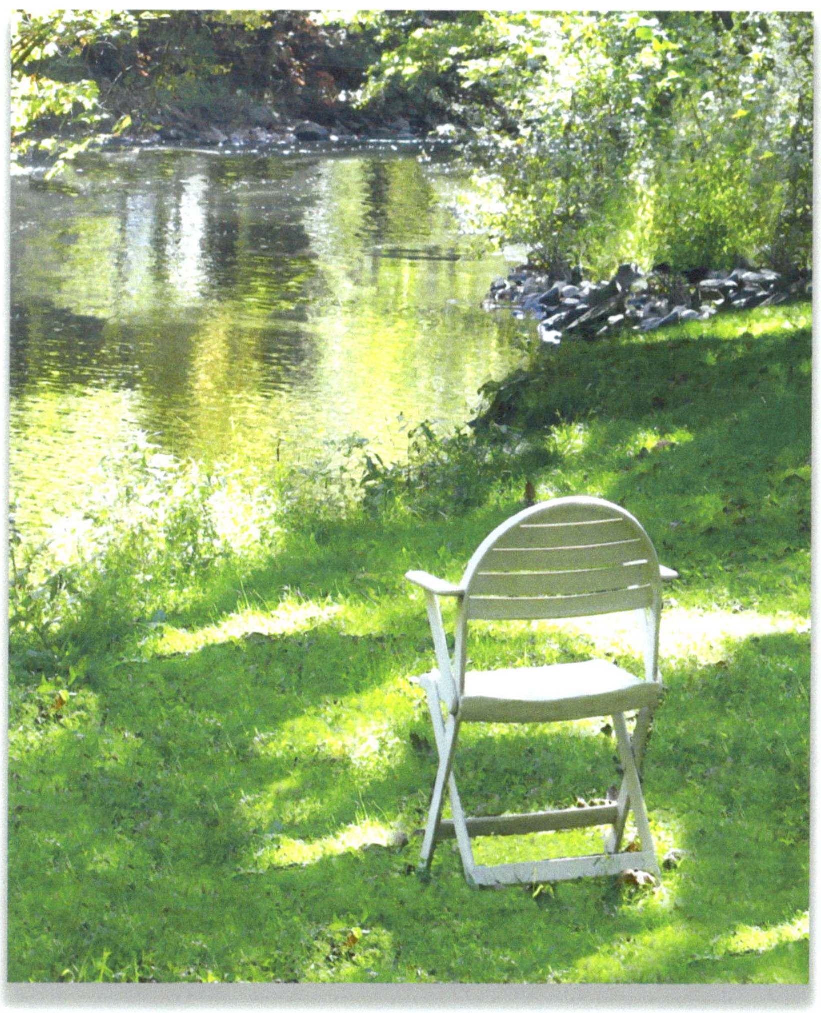

Take Time to PAUSE

Every successful journey, whether planned or unplanned, begins with a **Pause,** or a temporary stop. Taking this time allows you to assess your location, determine your destination and then plan how you'll get there.

Engaging in a healing journey may be a new adventure for you. However, with an open heart and mind, I can assure you that this will be a time of great change, growth and learning.

I encourage you to take the time, or PAUSE, to rest, be still and reflect. These are activities most of us don't have time for due to busy lives and sensory overload.

Through this healing journey, I urge you to be patient and compassionate with yourself. Let your open-hearted awareness and kindness guide your thoughts, feelings, choices and actions as you take this uncharted path toward self-discovery, healing and renewal.

Now, let's begin by learning about the most accessible and free healing tool on this planet...your breath.

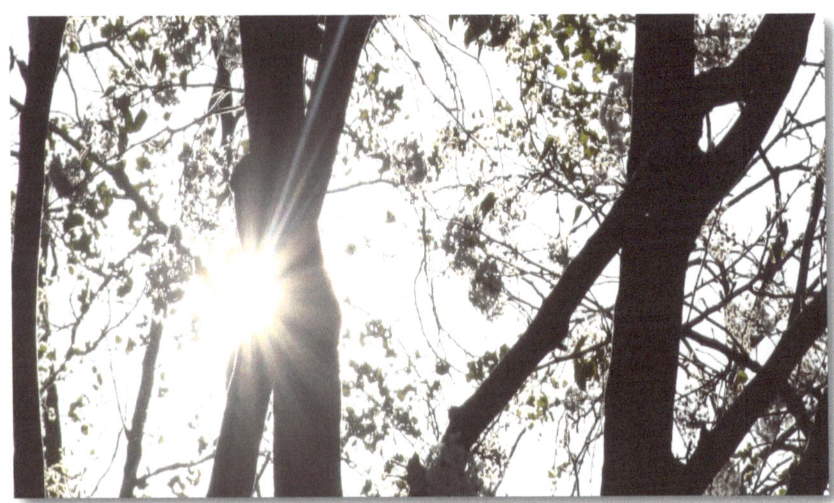

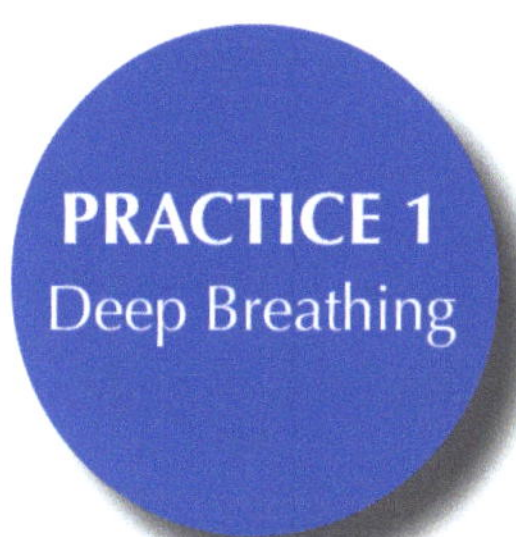

Learning to breathe deeply and with awareness can help restore your physical and emotional health in the following ways:

- Lowered blood pressure
- Increased energy
- Reduced anxiety and depression

Taking deep breaths relaxes your body and strengthens your immune system. Here are some deep breathing exercises to get you on the road to improved health. Practice focused breathing for five minutes every hour for optimum relaxation and healing.

Simple Deep Belly Breathing

1. While seated or laying down, place your hand on your belly.
2. Close your eyes and focus on your breath.
3. Breathe through your nose.
4. Inhale so that your belly elevates your hand.
5. Exhale until your hand is lowered.

Once this simple deep breathing method becomes natural, try the following deeper breathing techniques.

PAUSE Breathing Technique

1. Place your hands on your lap, to PAUSE in the moment.
2. Focus only on your breathing.
3. Deepen your relaxation by listening to the sound your body makes. Feel your belly and chest expand and contract. Notice the air coming in through your nose and out through your mouth....Just relax.
4. After five deep breaths, place one hand on your heart to initiate your body's natural anti-stress hormone, oxytocin.
5. Focus on your breath and nothing more as you ease into a more gentle PAUSE for five more breaths.

Peace and Calm Breathing Technique

1. Use simple deep breathing belly breaths.
2. Breathe in through your nose while envisioning the word 'Peace' in your mind. Hold for two counts and release through your mouth while envisioning the word 'Calm' in your mind.

Your Path to PEACE: Step 1

Practice the following exercises each day. Consider writing down any thoughts/feelings that arise. These notes will serve as trail markers on your healing journey.

Practice Breathing
- Set a timer and repeat deep breathing exercises throughout the day.
- Put your hand on your heart to connect with yourself and deepen your practice.

Change Your Mind with Affirmations
Affirmations are medicine for your mind when you truly connect with the words you are saying. Silently repeat these positive affirmations throughout the day to accelerate your healing journey.
- I am healing.
- Every day is a new beginning.
- My breath connects me to PEACE.

Honor Your Body
Your body allows you to experience ALL of life with its amazing design. Create a healing partnership with your body by mindfully thanking it (YES, THANKING IT) for making it possible to engage in this life adventure. Begin with your feet and move all the way up to your head, thanking each part of your body for helping you live and experience your life.

Imagine Your Even More Grateful Self
Focusing on gratitude is a powerful healing tool. Knowing what you **truly** appreciate and then appreciating it even more in your life, lifts your vitality. Create a list of all the goodness in your life, both present and past. This will bring you closer to a state of profound gratitude, elevating your spirit, inner peace and healing.

Your Thoughts

____

____

____

____

____

____

____

____

____

____

____

____

____

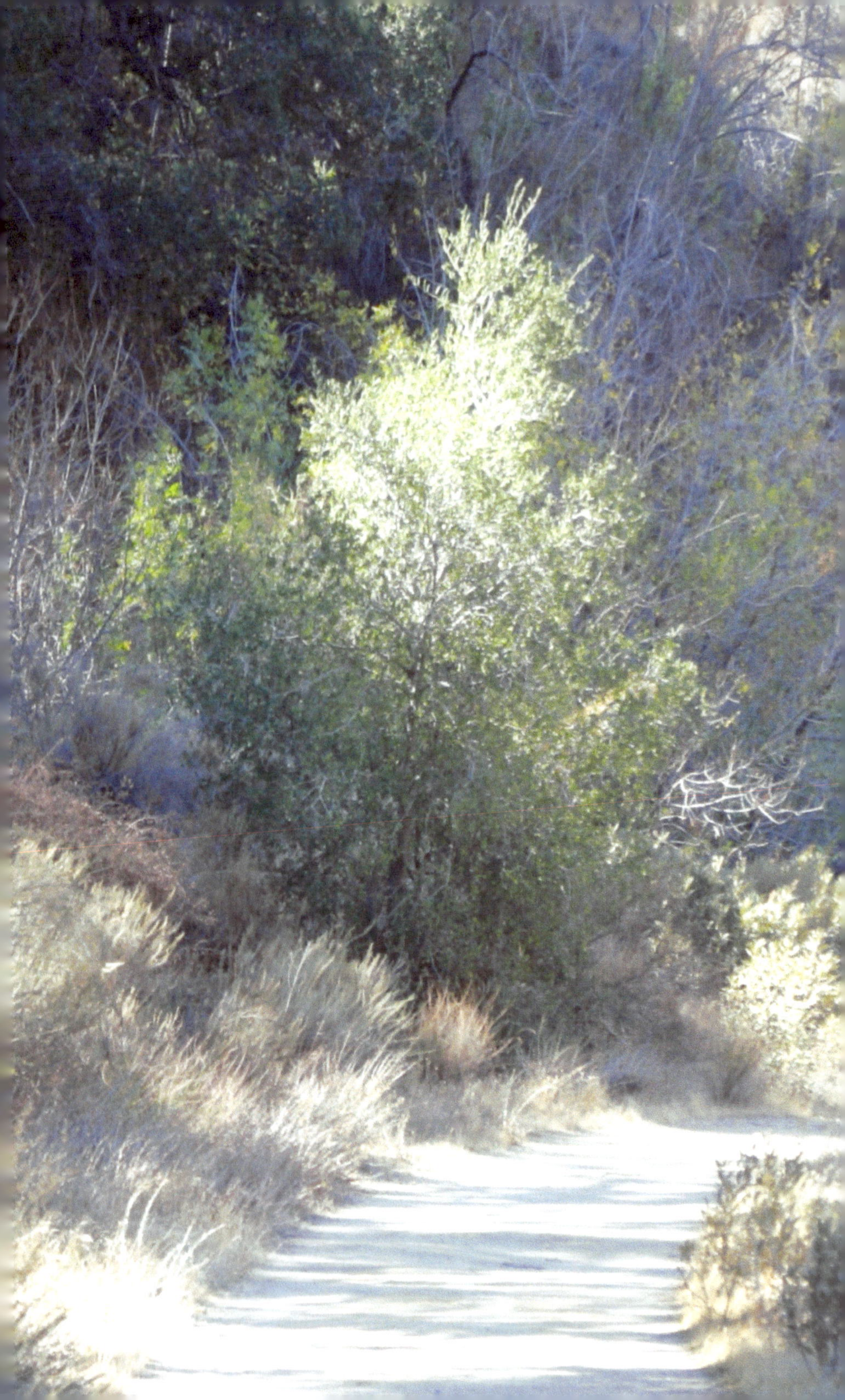

Your Time to EXPLORE

"In wisdom gathered over time, I have found that every experience is a form of exploration."

~Ansel Adams

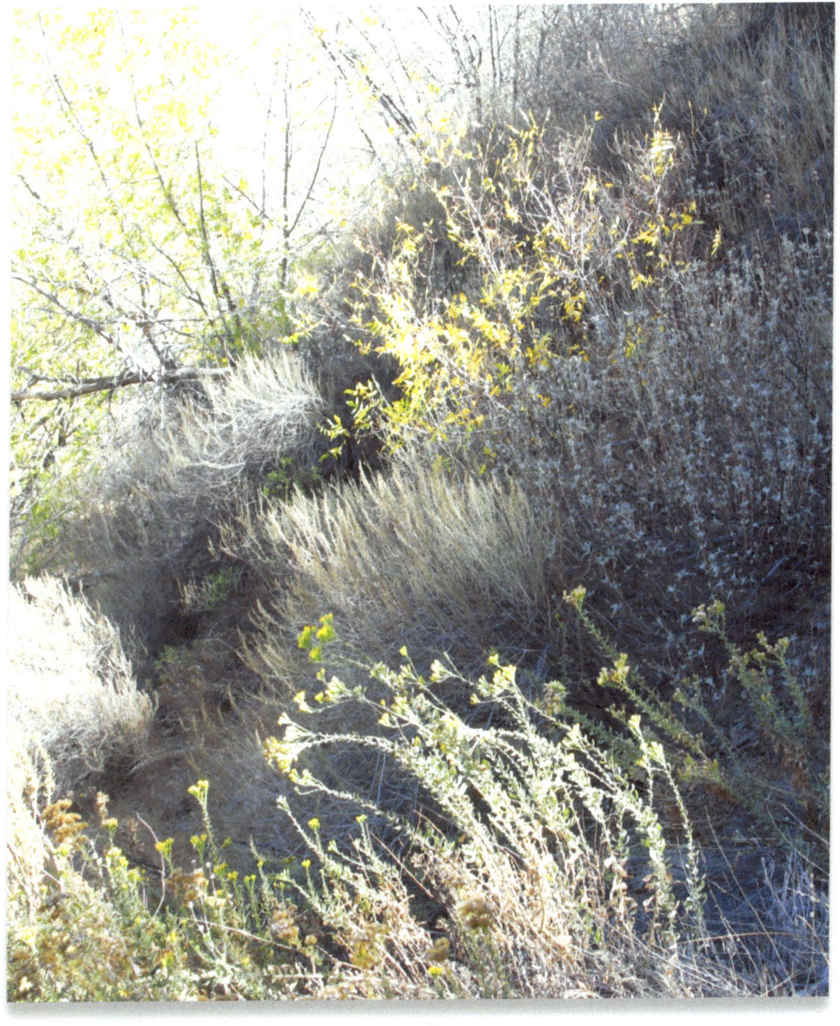

EXPLORE Your Body, Mind & Spirit

Your healing journey to inner PEACE started with a **Pause**. Remember to practice focused breathing so it becomes your automatic response to any stressors in your life.

In this section, we will **Explore** your body, mind and spirit with some simple questions to help make sure you are taking good care of yourself in daily life. Your answers will give you the insight to see if you need to make adjustments to your thoughts, attitudes or lifestyle for improved overall well-being.

When answering these questions, take note of any emotional or physical responses. Do you feel tension in your shoulders? Tightness in your chest? Do you feel sadness?

A strong positive response to any question indicates where you are doing just fine. Conversely, a strong negative response indicates where a change might be needed. Do not judge, simply be honest with yourself. This clarity is a big leap toward inner peace on your healing journey.

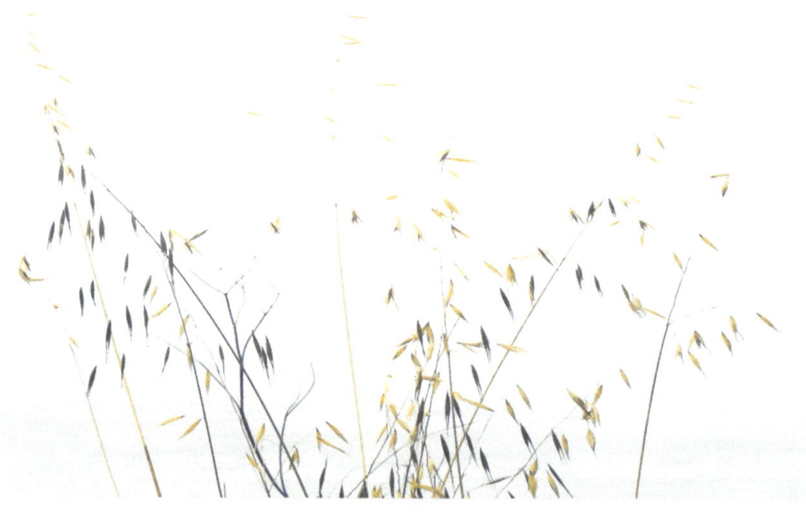

Your Body

1. Do you take good care of your body through healthy eating and exercise?
☐Yes ☐No   Why or why not?
____

2. Do you smile at yourself when you look in the mirror?
☐Yes ☐No   What do you see?______________________

3. Do you appreciate everything your AMAZING body can do?
☐Yes ☐No   What's the most amazing?______________

4. Do you give your body the rest it needs to recharge?
☐Yes ☐No   What could you do better?______________

Your Mind

1. Do you give your mind 'down' time to sit quietly?
☐Yes ☐No   Why or why not?______________________

2. Do you challenge your behaviors that don't serve you?
☐Yes ☐No What would you change?______________

3. Do you feel like you're drowning in overwhelm?
☐Yes ☐No   What's the source?______________________

Your Spirit

1. Do you engage in activities that make life more fun?
☐Yes ☐No   Why or why not?______________________

2. Do you connect with others when you need support?
☐Yes ☐No   Why or why not?______________________

3. Can you list 10 things for which you are deeply grateful?
☐Yes ☐No   List them on 'Your Thoughts' (page 15).

4. Are you usually kind to yourself and others?
☐Yes ☐No   Why or why not?______________________

5. Do you have a positive impact on those around you?
☐Yes ☐No   Why or why not?______________________

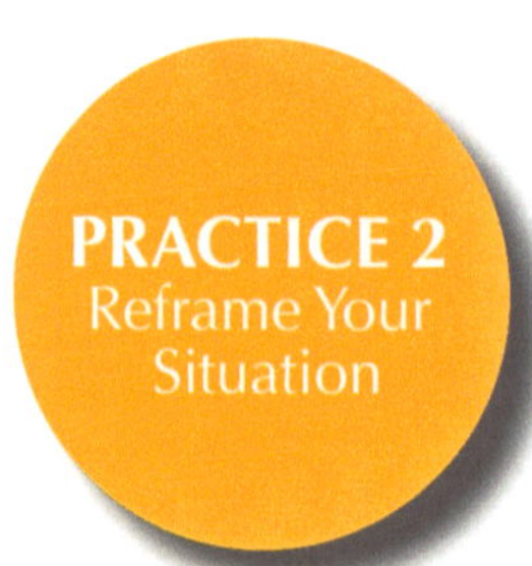

Cognitive reframing is a technique that helps you pivot from feeling out of control to clear-minded, problem-solving thinking. With consistent practice, cognitive reframing will help you:

- Shift your thinking patterns from negative to positive.
- Remove negative thoughts that prevent you from achieving your full potential.
- Change the way you cope with stressful events.
- Improve the quality of your life and relationships.

Use the 'Practice Reframing' worksheet on the next page to identify your challenges and negative thoughts. Then reframe your situation using the following tips.

1. Reframe your challenges as *"opportunities to learn & grow,"* instead of as *"obstacles."*
2. Reframe *"I can't..."* with *"I wonder how I can..."*
3. Reframe *"Ugh, I have to..."* with *"Yay, I'm able to..."*
4. Reframe *"This will never happen."* with *"Anything is possible."*
5. Reframe your thinking to the *best-case scenario* instead of *worst-case scenario.*

For some, thinking positive takes a bit more effort. By bringing awareness to your thoughts AND making a conscious commitment to this reframing practice, you'll be rewarded with new perspectives and insights.

If you get stuck in a negative thinking pattern after attempting to reframe your situation, go back to Step 1 to PAUSE and practice deep breathing. Also, immerse yourself in the nature photos throughout this guide. They will help you connect with the beauty of life. When you are ready, go back to the reframing practice. Notice the difference a PAUSE can make toward the goal of achieving PEACE!

Practice Reframing

Your Challenge	Your Negative Thought	Reframe Your Situation to a More Productive Thought
Two examples. 1. I can't get ahead.	Life isn't fair. Things go wrong a lot.	Wow, this challenge is really teaching me how to overcome obstacles.
2. Life is over-whelming most of the time.	I can't believe I'm sick. I have SO MUCH to do.	My body really knew I needed to slow down and rest.

Your Path to PEACE: Step 2

Practice the following exercises each day. Consider writing down your thoughts/feelings that arise. These notes will serve as trail markers on your healing journey.

Practice Reframing
- Set your default thinking to the best-case scenario.
- If you experience a challenge, don't panic. Instead, think of solutions and write them down.
- Reframe a setback as an opportunity to grow and learn.

Change Your Mind with Affirmations
Affirmations are medicine for your mind when you truly connect with the words you are saying. Silently repeat these positive affirmations throughout the day to accelerate your healing journey.
- Forgiveness releases me from anger.
- I grow from my experiences and struggles.
- My struggles lead to inner strength and self-awareness.

Replenish Your Body
More than 50 percent of your body is made of water. Water flushes body waste through sweat and urine, helps with digestion and delivers oxygen to all parts of your body. Drinking water helps restore balance in your body and removes toxins. When possible, drink at least a half gallon of water (64 fluid ounces) daily to promote a healthier body. Add lemon or lime for extra vitamin C.

Imagine Your Stronger Self
Bringing awareness to your inner strength is an effective tool toward inner peace and healing. Create a list of challenges you've already overcome and your strengths it took to do so. (Yes, we ALL have inner strength.)

Your Thoughts

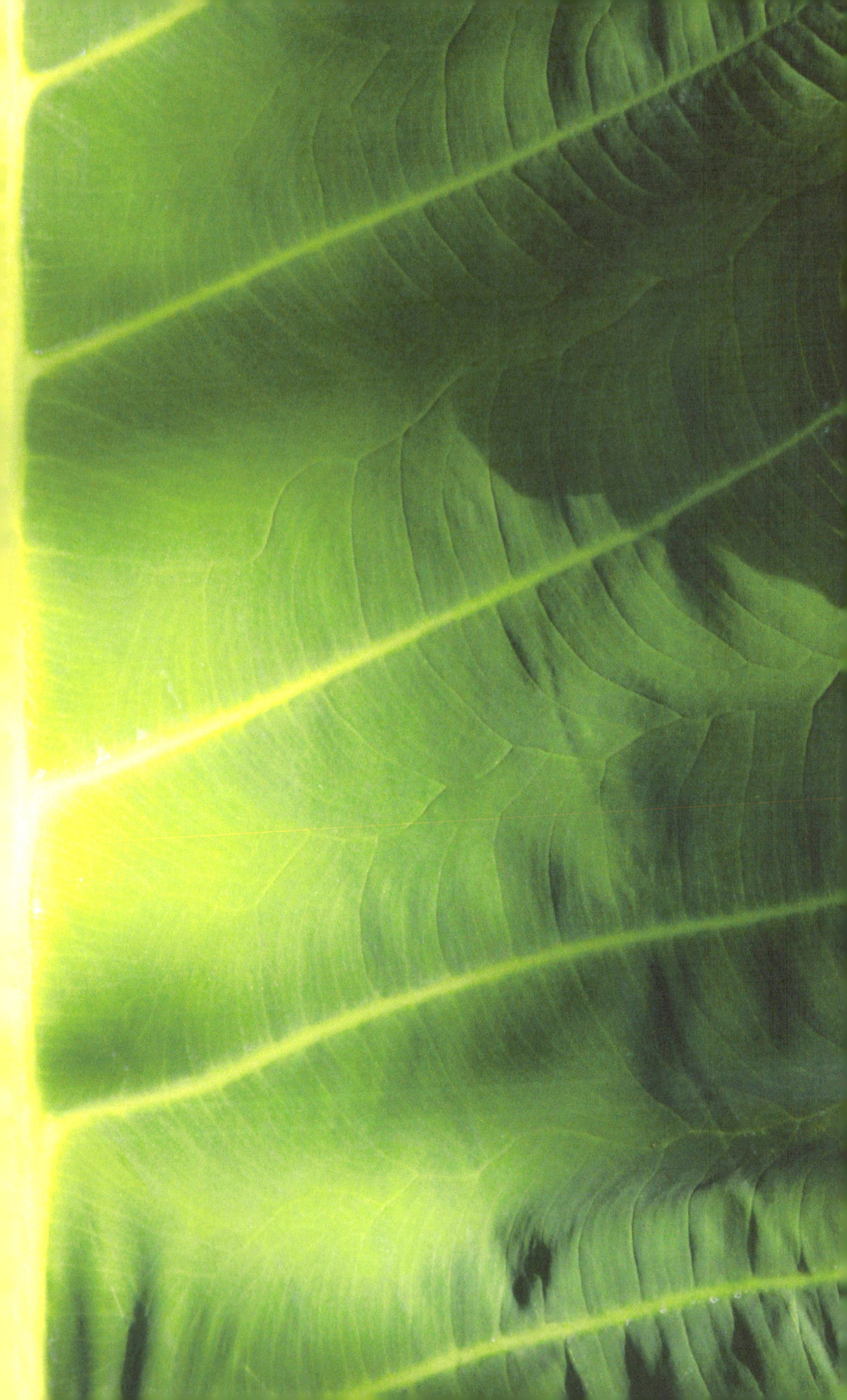

Your Time to ALIGN

"What is necessary to change a person is to change his awareness of himself."

~Abraham Maslow

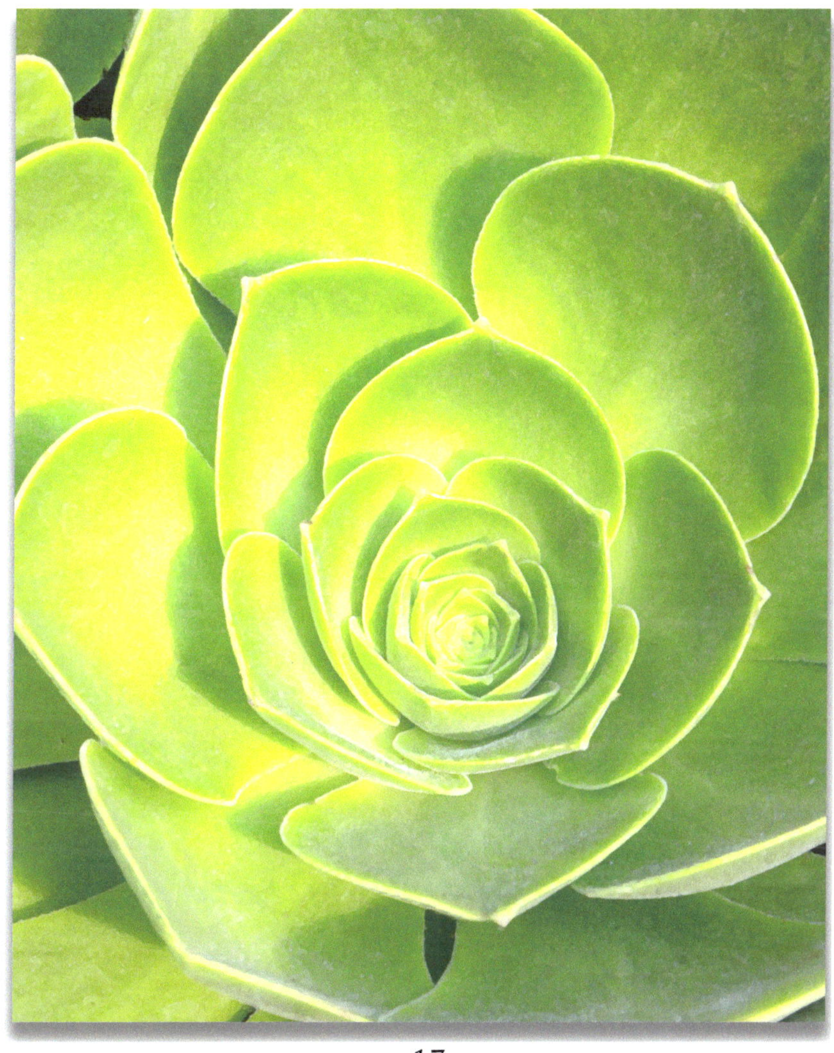

ALIGN Your Body, Mind and Spirit

So far your path to inner PEACE has consisted of **Pausing** and **Exploring.** In this section, we will focus on **Aligning** your body, mind and spirit.

It's like a balancing act. When one part of you is out of alignment, you become unbalanced. This in turn affects your physical and emotional health.

For balanced well-being, it is important to know if you're taking good care of your body, mind and spirit on a daily basis. Identifying your personal values, priorities, hopes and dreams is a lens to clarify if you're living a life that's aligned with your whole self.

To help you move toward alignment, I have included a variety of questions, some easy and some tough, so you can pinpoint where you might be off balance.

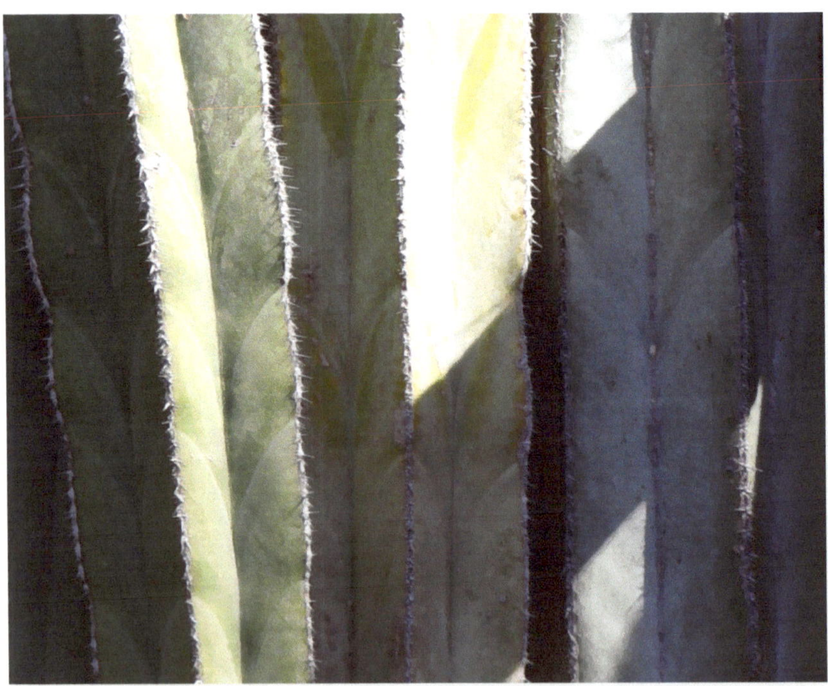

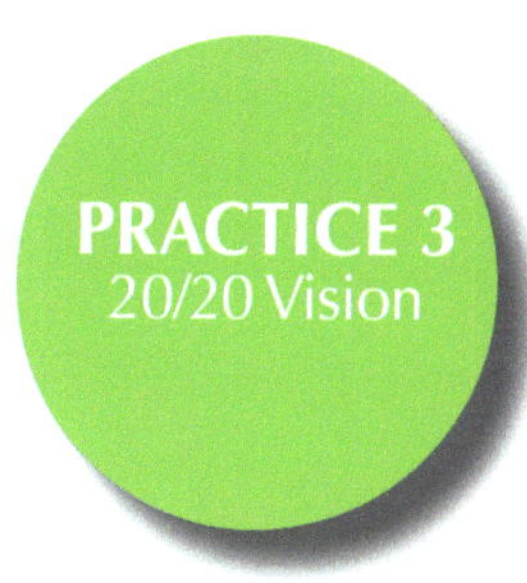

Aligning your body, mind and spirit is a key step in your healing journey. To move forward, you need to see yourself objectively and truthfully.

One way to do this is to put on imaginary 20/20 perfect vision glasses. With perfect vision, you can see your strengths, weaknesses, challenges and opportunities, more clearly and honestly.

Wearing your perfect vision glasses, answer the questions on pages 20-21. They will help you identify where you are, how you got here and what you must do to move ahead on your healing journey. Consider all your options and enjoy your clarity. Here are some things you may discover.

Your Body
- Identify ways you are already taking good care of your body.
- Uncover lifestyle behaviors you can make or change to take better care of your body.

Your Mind
- Tap into your natural ability to accelerate your emotional and physical healing.
- Identify burdens, judgments and negative thoughts that interfere with your emotional and physical healing.

Your Spirit
- Discover what brings you joy and gratitude.
- Expose any limiting beliefs you put on yourself that may be preventing you from having fun or appreciating all that you DO have.
- Establish a deeper connection with your joyful heart.

May you find even more balance to steady you on your path.

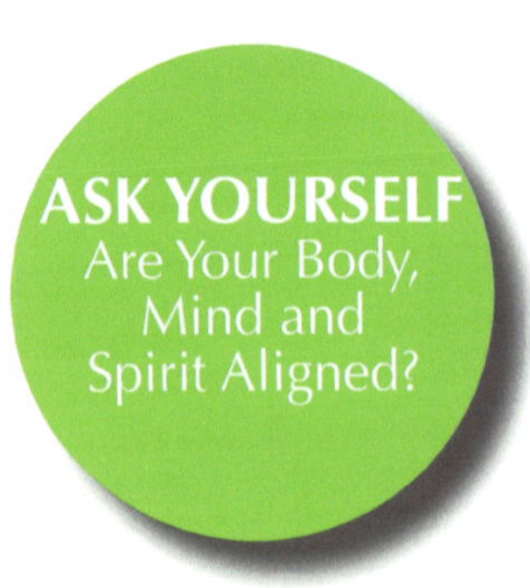

Your Body

1. Why is having a healthy body important to you?

2. What consistent practices do you use to support your healthy body?

3. What small step can you take today to move toward an even healthier body? (For example: Drink lots of water to cleanse the inside of your body!)

4. Do you value your healthy body as an important asset to your life experience?

5. List three kind words to say to your body right now.

Your Mind

1. Are you carrying burdens that might be affecting your mood?

2. Have you considered ways to solve your burdens?

3. Are you holding negative judgments about yourself or others? (For example: Not being 'good enough'.) If so, why?

4. Is there anyone in your life, past or present, whom you can forgive for causing you hurt and pain?
(Note: Forgiveness is a very effective healing balm.)

5. Do you have negative thinking patterns or unhealthy habits that might cause stress, anxiety or depression? (For example: worrying.)

Your Mind

6. Have you considered learning about mindfulness or meditation to help with stress?

7. What do you like most about yourself?

8. What are your greatest strengths and innate gifts?

9. For what or whom are you deeply grateful? Why?

Your Spirit

1. Do you allow yourself to have fun? How often?

2. How do you relax? How often?

3. How can you include more self-care practices into your life? What would you include?

4. Do you feel supported or connected to anyone who 'has your back'?

5. Do you help others - friends, family, co-workers or strangers - in a way that creates self-worth?

6. What hopes and dreams do you wish for? Do you have plans to make them a reality?

7. What do you value most in your life and why? How does this important value enhance your existence?

Your Path to PEACE: Step 3

Practice the following exercises on a regular basis. Consider writing down any thoughts/feelings that arise. These notes will serve as trail markers on your healing journey.

Practice Alignment
- Let go of all negative thoughts and judgments.
- Free yourself to think of experiences that make you feel happy, worthy, joyful, peaceful and strong.
- Use your heart as a compass to know if you're moving in the right direction. Your heart KNOWS what feels right.

Change Your Mind with Affirmations
Affirmations are medicine for your mind when you truly connect with the words you are saying. Silently repeat these positive affirmations throughout the day to accelerate your healing journey.
- My body, mind and spirit are cultivating more balance.
- I am grateful to my body for the healing it is doing.
- I am willing to take even better care of my body.

Accept Your Body
Living with acceptance for your body 'as is' creates the opportunity to love yourself (and your life) even more. This love and acceptance serve as the foundation for you to think clearly and consider all your options to initiate any changes that will improve your health and well-being. No matter what your age - like the seasons, we are always changing whether we want to or not.

Imagine Your Healthier Self
Visualization is such an effective healing tool. Take the time to visualize your healthier self. Imagine all the healthy habits you're practicing to maintain your balance. Write down the fun activities you'll be doing as you move toward a healthier and more vibrant you.

Your Thoughts

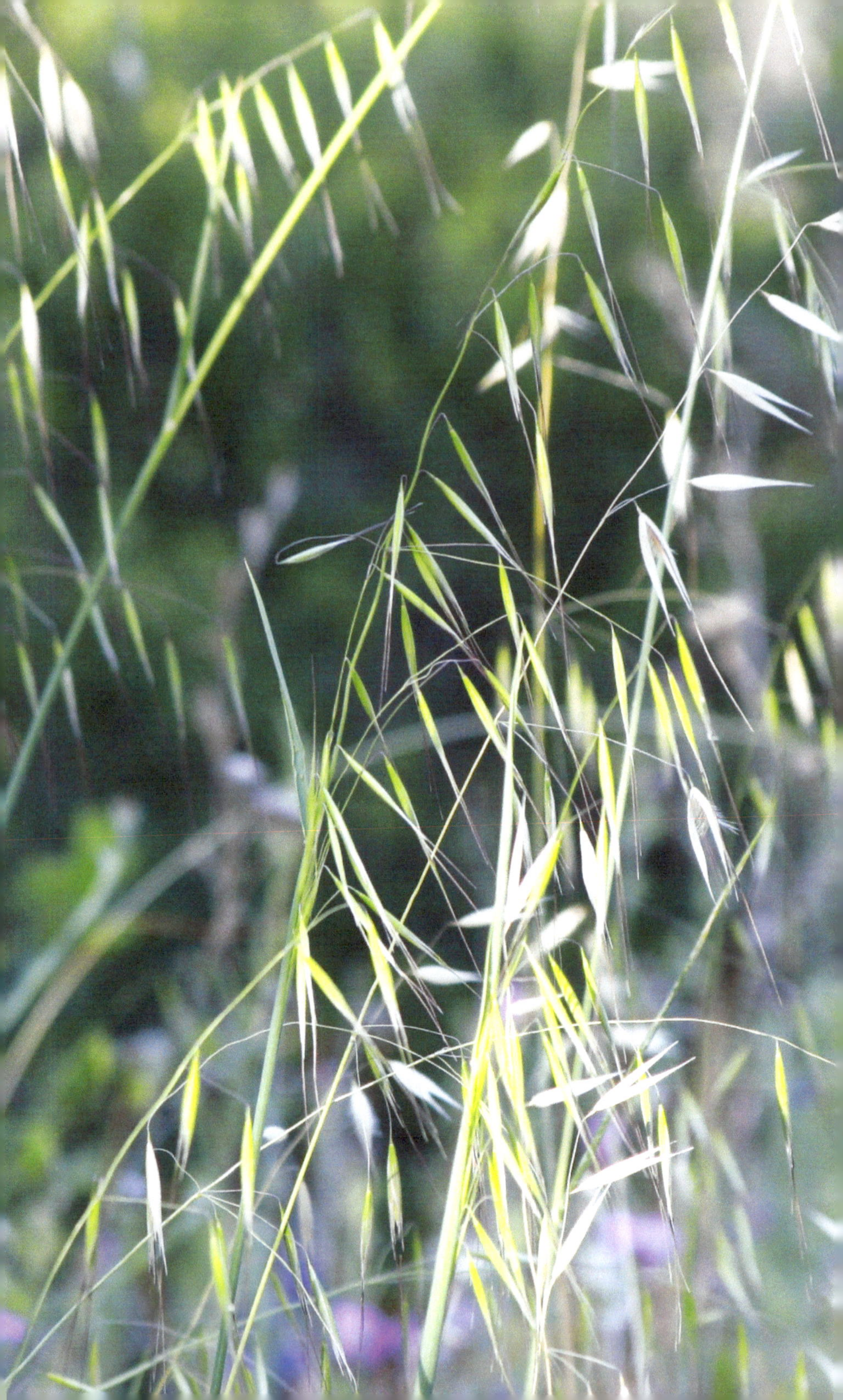

Your Time to CHOOSE

"There are two primary choices in life:
accept conditions as they exist, or accept the
responsibility for changing them."

~Denis Waitley

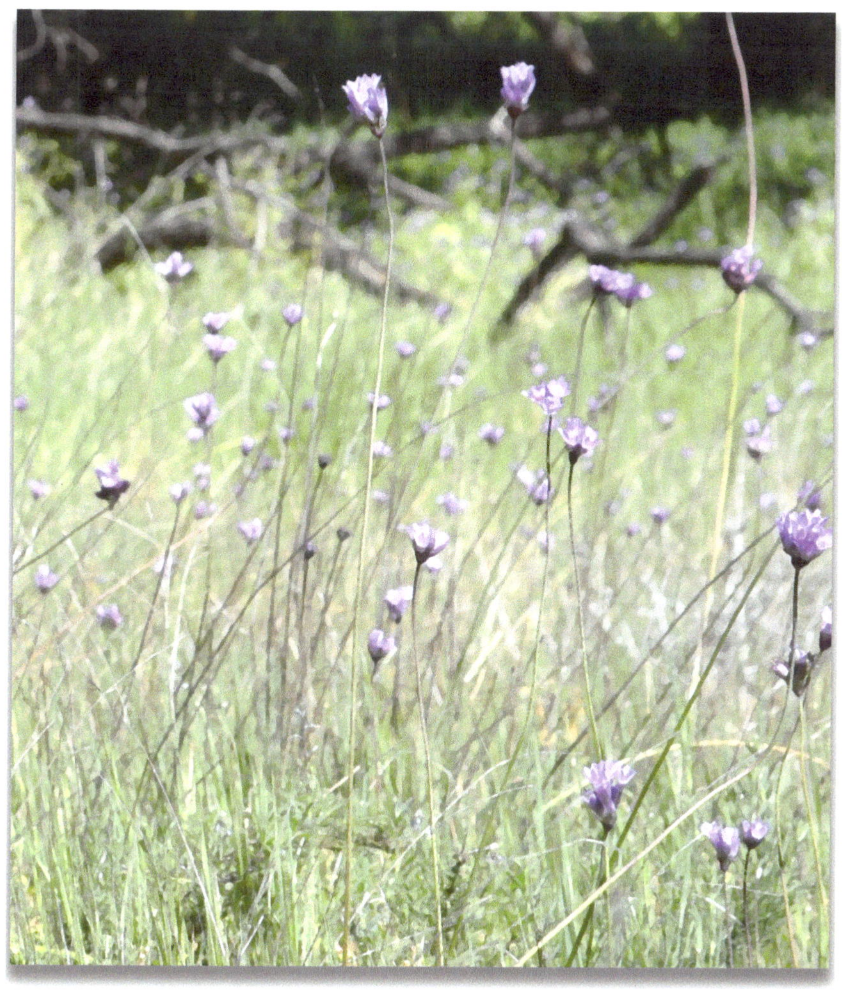

CHOOSE What's Best for You

At this point, you've done a lot of good work to know yourself even more. After completing the **Pausing**, **Exploring**, and **Aligning** sections, you're getting closer to reaching more Inner PEACE. The next step, making conscious **Choices**, often gets lost in the everyday busyness, activities and obligations of life.

It's important to note that every Choice you make has an effect on your body, mind and spirit, as well as on the people around you. Some of your choices may cause stress, anxiety and despair, while others provide joy, inner peace and healing.

The goal of this section is to help you bring more awareness to the Choices you make as you move forward in your journey to improved health and happiness. Believe it or not, even your thoughts are a choice.

With any choice you make, ask yourself these questions.
- *Is this choice loving toward myself?*
- *Is this choice laying the groundwork for sustained health and vitality?*
- *Is this choice aligned with my hopes and dreams?*

Take the time to consider how you'll feel AFTER the choice(s) you're about to make. For example, how will you feel after choosing to have a healthy snack vs. something not so healthy?

If for some reason you find yourself making choices that are not aligned with your well-being, get curious and consider these questions.
- *Why am I choosing this when I KNOW it doesn't support my well-being?*
- *What other choice can I make that ALIGNS with my well-being, my long-term goals and my desires?*

What if things happened for you, not against you.

You have the freedom to take ownership of, and be in a healthy relationship with your choices, beliefs, actions and thoughts.
For example, if you made a mistake in the past (like we ALL have), you can make the choice to forgive yourself. If something feels overwhelming to you, you can make the choice to take deep breaths to signal your nervous system into the rest and relaxation response. For your higher level of well-being, consider making the choices that nourish your body, mind and soul.

You *know* what choices create your more meaningful life.
You *can* figure out or learn the necessary steps to fulfill your dreams.
You *can* create more inner peace for yourself and those around you.
Honestly, you are so much stronger than you know.

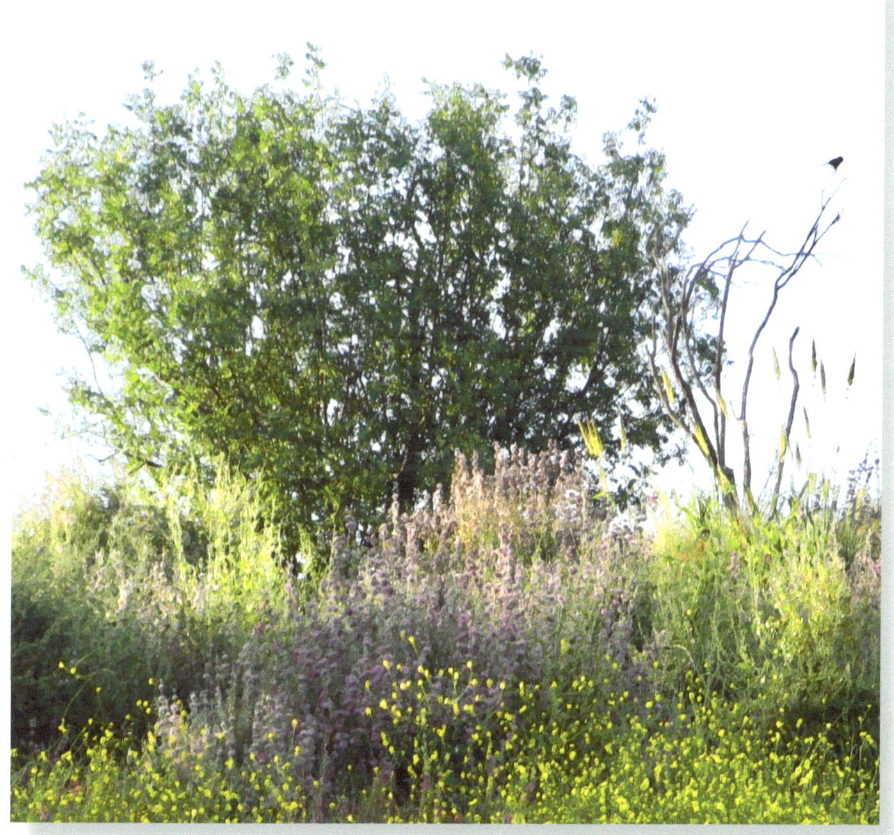

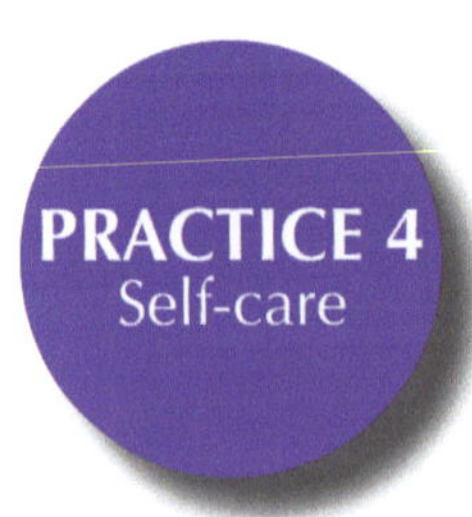

Self-care means taking proper care of yourself in a way that nurtures your well-being. There are numerous benefits of self-care, including:

- Lower anxiety
- More energy
- Increased confidence
- Improved quality of life

Here are some ways to start practicing self-care whatever your situation.

Body self-care

Food. Limit fats and sugar. Eat more vegetables and fruits to help your body take care of itself. Keep a food journal to track what and when you eat. If you are a stress eater, find healthy alternatives.

Water. Keep your body hydrated to flush out toxins. Aim to drink 64 ounces of water each day. Supplement water with a relaxing time to drink herbal tea.

Exercise. Start with a brisk walk three days a week for 30 minutes. If you're unable to walk, do what my wheelchair-bound neighbor does; lift weights or do chair yoga!

Sleep. Most people need eight hours of sleep each night. Practice good sleep hygiene. Go to bed and wake up the same time each day, skip caffeine in the afternoon and evening, create a relaxing pre-sleep ritual, and say good night to your smart phone, computer and television at least a half hour before bed.

Mind self-care

Find PEACE. Practice the skills you've learned to create inner PEACE. This includes Pausing (breathing) and Exploring (using the reframing techniques and practicing a more positive projected outcome).

Forgive. Let go of negative experiences. Be grateful for all the goodness in your life, from the simple to the amazing. This is a wonderful gift to give yourself.

Mind self-care

Unplug. Spend a day without social media and email. Go to a park and read. Listen to your favorite music. Start writing whatever comes to mind in a journal.

Be Social. Healthy relationships are an important part of good physical and mental health. Work on developing or strengthening relationships with friends or family that support your well-being.

Spirit self-care

Meditate/Pray Find deep relaxation and connection to a universal higher power if that feels right to you.

Find purpose. Using the techniques you've learned in this guide, think about your accomplishments (small and big). How can you build on them? For example: If you overcame a tremendous challenge, you can teach others to do the same.

Volunteer. Find a cause that you are interested in and volunteer your time. Even if it's just a couple hours a month, it will make you feel good and give you a sense of purpose.

Spend time in nature. Find peace in nature's amazing beauty.

Note: If you notice that you continue to make choices that do not align with your well-being, dig a bit deeper. You might want to consider getting insight from a therapist, coach, trusted friend, self-help book or website. You can also take online self-help classes to help you understand yourself even better. A good place to start is *Udemy.com*.

Choose and commit to a number of self-care practices for a week. Continue increasing your practices to create lifelong, healthy habits and elevated well-being.

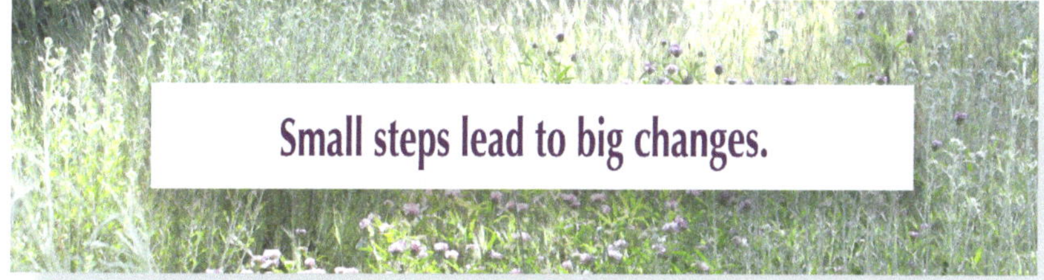

Your Path to PEACE: Step 4

Practice the following exercises regularly. Consider writing down your thoughts/feelings that arise. These notes will serve as trail markers on your healing journey. Keep moving forward.

Practice Self-Care
- Choose and begin one restorative and fun activity for your heart and soul. Schedule this for at least 15 minutes daily.
- Bring more awareness to your choices. Celebrate your choices that support your well-being and explore choices that don't align with your health by keeping a daily journal.

Change Your Mind with Affirmations
Affirmations are medicine for your mind when you truly connect with the words. Silently repeat these positive affirmations throughout the day to accelerate your healing journey.
- I am free to choose my attitude of gratitude.
- I am alive with unlimited possibilities.
- I make choices to support my well-being and vitality.

Recharge Your Body
The food choices you make and put into your body are part of the fuel that ignites health and healing. Take the time to learn more about healthy eating habits and recipes that will support your immune system and healthier body.

Imagine Your Happier Self
Happiness fosters peace and peace brings health and vitality. Close your eyes and imagine your future happier self. What are you doing? How do you feel? Where are you? What do you see? In detail, write down this picture of your happier self on the next page and use as a guide for cultivating and tending your even more joyful self.

Your Thoughts

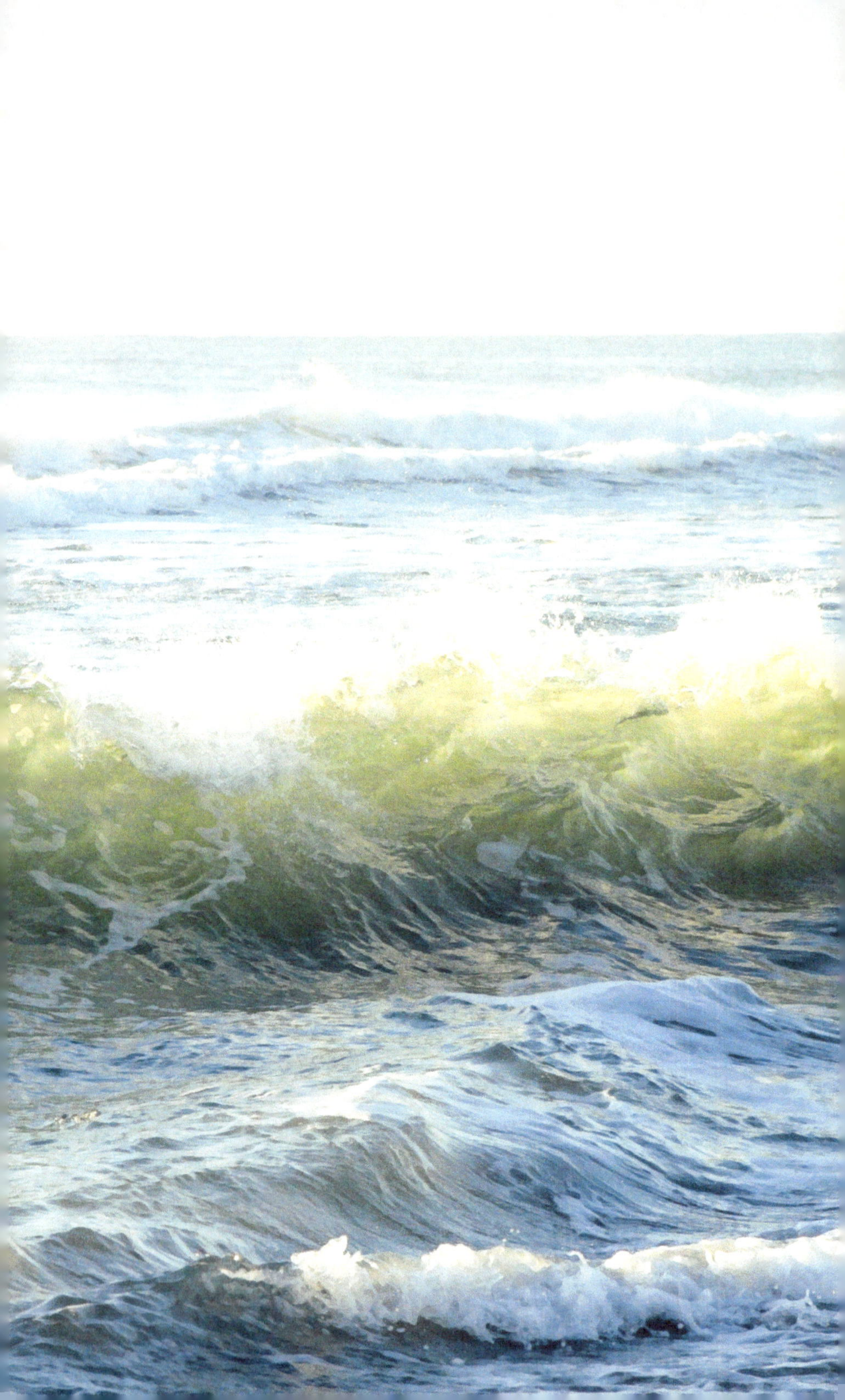

Your Time to EXPERIENCE

"Our greatness lies not so much in being able to
remake the world, but being able to
remake ourselves."

~Mahatma Gandhi

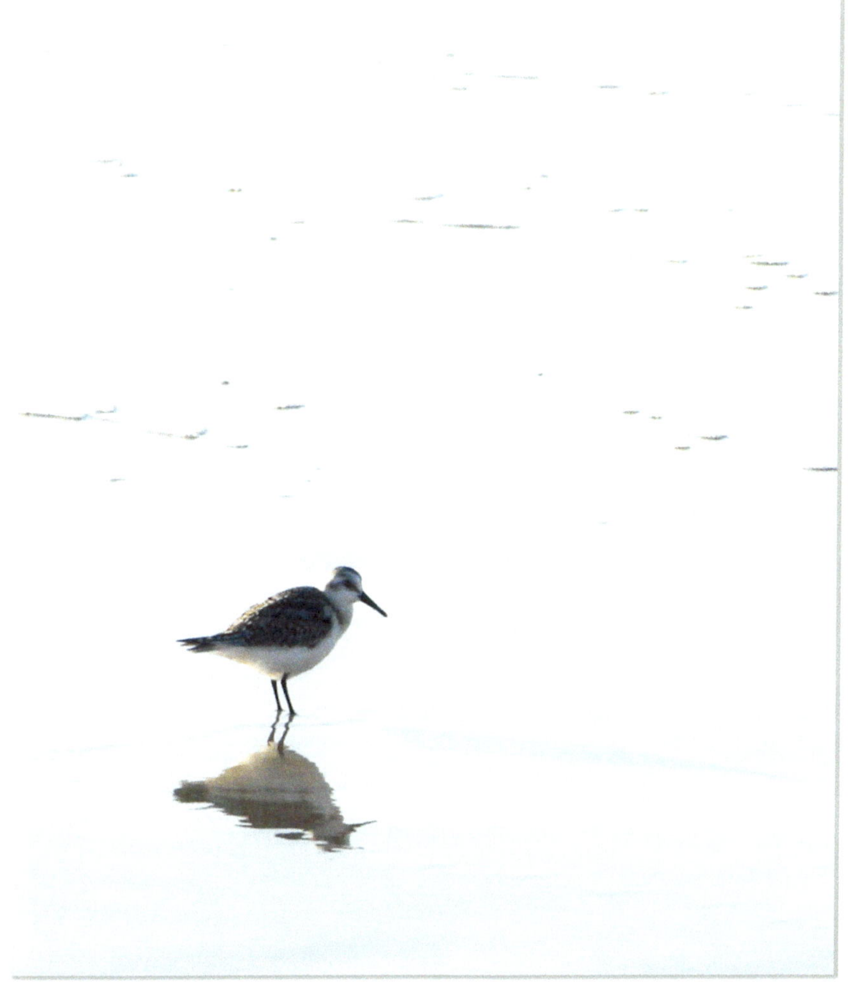

EXPERIENCE the New You!

Fully experiencing your life is to fully express your authentic self to the world. Be the song of your loving heart, your balanced body, mind and spirit…as best you can.

To review your healing journey, you've **Paused** to reflect on the things that are important to you, you've **Explored** and brought awareness in order to **Align** with your **Choices**, and learned what to do in case your choices aren't supporting your well-being.

Hopefully, you've used this valuable time to reflect on your body, mind and spirit. I hope you've been honest with yourself and are committed to continuing your healthy and vibrant journey forward. Finally, it's time to **Experience** the new you.

Did you know your chances of being born are one in 400 trillion? You were born for a reason and you have a greater purpose…to be your best self and then to bring your best self, your gifts and your kindness out into the world. (Not always easy, I know.)

When you are able, be sure to spend time in nature and use your senses. Look at the ever-changing sky, flowing streams and twinkling stars. Feel the whispering winds, sandy beaches and warm sun. Smell the fresh flowers and fresh-cut grass. Taste the juicy fruits and hearty vegetables. Nature is an amazing paradise…where you can always go to find PEACE. Remember, each day really is a brand new beginning.

Take care dear friend and continue the steps to your improved health - body, mind and spirit - as you engage in the rest of your amazing journey. I'll be thinking of you.

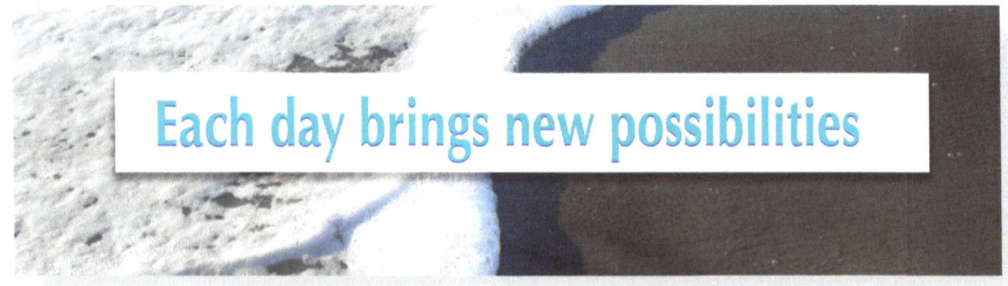

It's goal time.
It is important to set goals for yourself so you have things to look forward to. This is what makes life all the more exciting, meaningful and fun.

While setting goals gives you forward momentum, it is so important to first honor where you are right now. Honor this moment, as the present is all we truly have. As you learned, being appreciative of the present allows you to fully embrace yourself and your life right now. This is vital for your current well-being and an excellent starting point when setting goals. Keep in mind, we are all a work in progress learning from our experiences.

Before you set goals, please be sure to acknowledge the strides you've already made. This will strengthen your will to find solutions and keep moving should you stumble across any future roadblocks.

In order to achieve any goal, I suggest using the S.M.A.R.T. goal-setting method. This is a great method to keep your goals realistic so that you don't get overwhelmed with the details.

- **S.** **Specific.** What goal do you want to accomplish?
- **M.** **Measureable.** How will you know when you reach your goal?
- **A.** **Attainable.** Do you have the ability to accomplish it?
- **R.** **Realistic.** Is this a realistic goal for you?
- **T.** **Timely.** When can you achieve your goal?

Write down ALL your past achievements and use them as evidence that you have the capacity to achieve your aspirations. Refer to these jottings for momentum to keep you going. Write the 'Whys' (intentions) of your goals and use as motivation to keep you focused and moving forward. You so got this! Safe travels, my friend. Enjoy your journey.

Your Path to PEACE: Step 5

Practice the following exercises regularly. Consider writing down any thoughts/feelings that arise. Keep moving forward.

Practice the New You
- Write down S.M.A.R.T. goals that will move you forward as you forge ahead toward a happier, healthier, more peaceful, confident...YOU.
- Write down the Whys or intentions of attaining your goals and the positive outcomes you're anticipating.

Change Your Mind with Affirmations
Affirmations are medicine for your mind when you truly connect with the words. Silently repeat these positive affirmations throughout the day to accelerate your healing journey.
- Small goals keep me moving forward to more joy.
- Life offers me the opportunity to learn and grow.
- I am moving in the right direction.

Heal Your Body
Your AMAZING body is designed to heal and you ARE healing in more ways than you can ever imagine. Even if you might be experiencing pain at this moment - please know your body is trying its very best to help you heal. Remember to nourish your body with healthy food and visualize your body healing...because it really does heal.

Imagine Your More Loving Self
There is no greater life force than love. Close your eyes and imagine your future, more loving self. What kind words are you offering yourself and others? What gratitude are you feeling when looking in the mirror at your miraculous body? In detail, write down this picture of your loving self on the next page and use as a guide for being your radiant and delightful healing self - moving forward with compassion and inner peace.

Your Thoughts

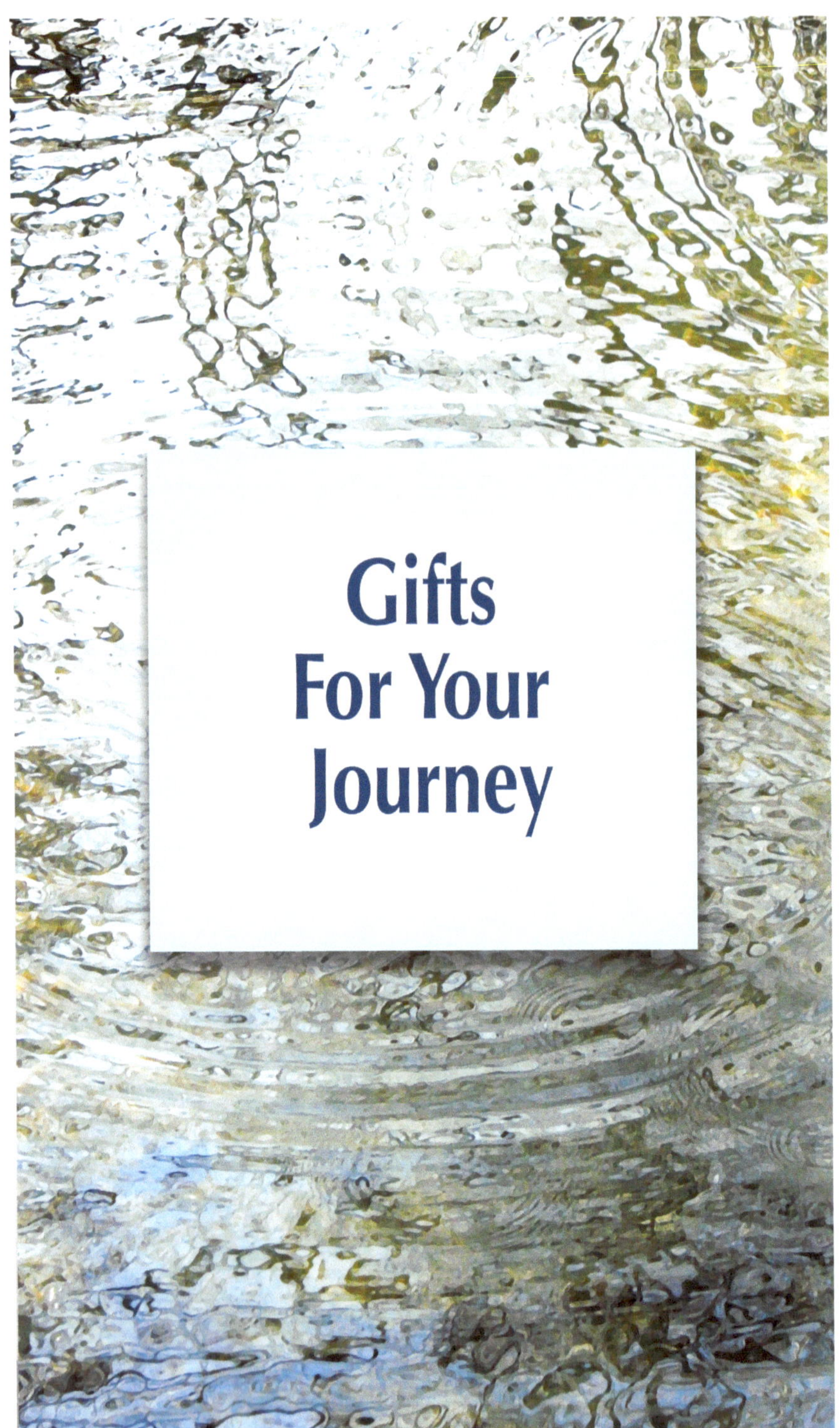
Gifts
For Your
Journey

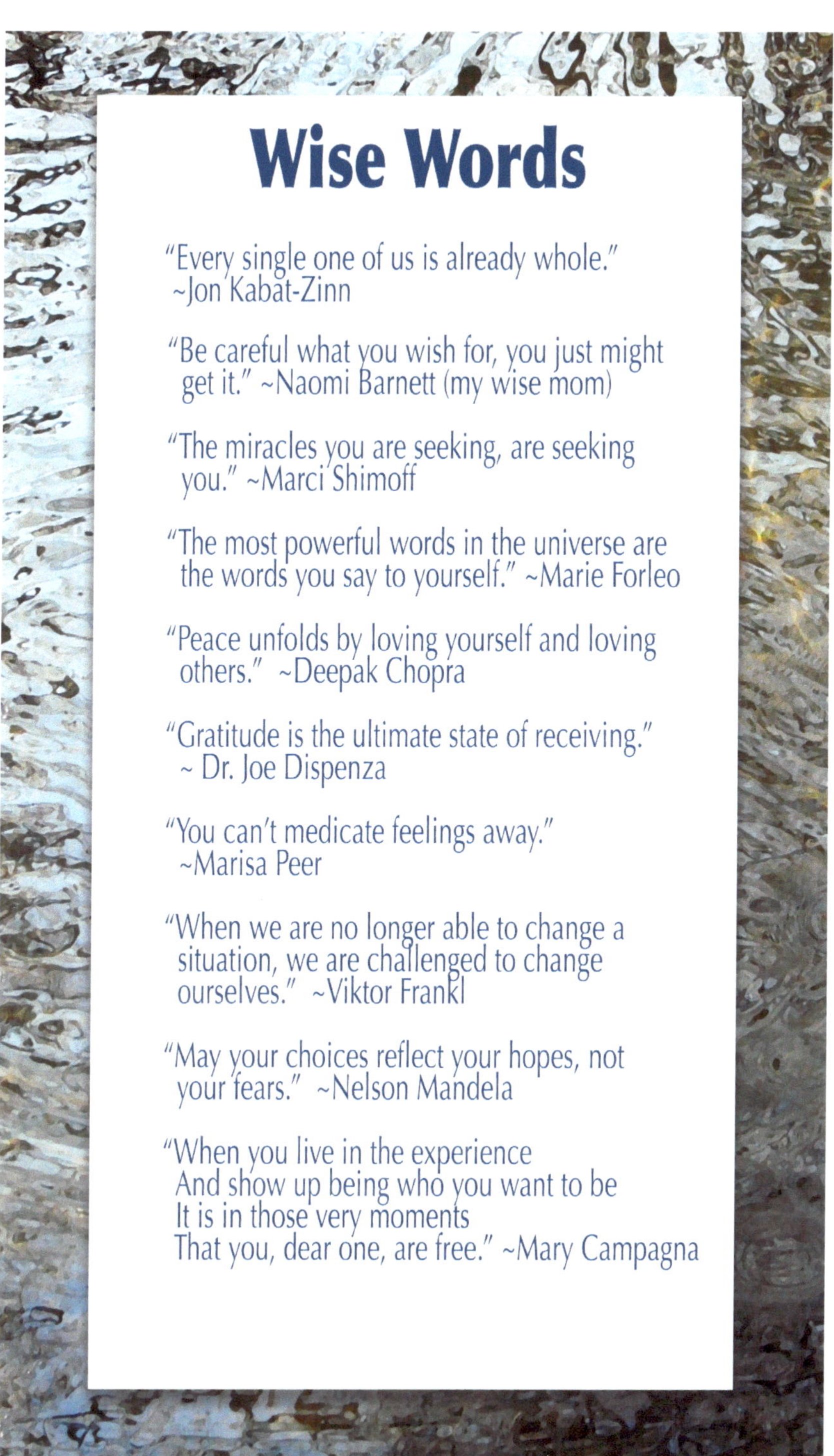

Wise Words

"Every single one of us is already whole."
~Jon Kabat-Zinn

"Be careful what you wish for, you just might
get it." ~Naomi Barnett (my wise mom)

"The miracles you are seeking, are seeking
you." ~Marci Shimoff

"The most powerful words in the universe are
the words you say to yourself." ~Marie Forleo

"Peace unfolds by loving yourself and loving
others." ~Deepak Chopra

"Gratitude is the ultimate state of receiving."
~ Dr. Joe Dispenza

"You can't medicate feelings away."
~Marisa Peer

"When we are no longer able to change a
situation, we are challenged to change
ourselves." ~Viktor Frankl

"May your choices reflect your hopes, not
your fears." ~Nelson Mandela

"When you live in the experience
And show up being who you want to be
It is in those very moments
That you, dear one, are free." ~Mary Campagna

A Cup of Comfort

Whether or not you believe in miracles, here is a true story I want to share. It happened to me in September 2019 while visiting my sister, who lives near the ocean.

It took me a long time to believe in miracles. Although everyone around me saw them, I did not. People who loved me would point out all the miracles they saw happen to me or happened to them. Despite the obvious synchronicities and their efforts to convince me, I did not believe the universe had my back. You see, having lost my parents to cancer while they were quite vibrant in their late 50's and also witnessing their pain and suffering - I was skeptical and soooo angry at life.

Spending time with my sister over the years, she would randomly find a penny or more and declared that for her, every time she found money, she perceived each cent as the universe sending her a message that she had unseen help. And so from time to time when my sister had justified worries, inevitably she would find pennies and KNEW everything would be ok...and it **always** was.

Later in my life, putting aside my anger, I opened my heart and adapted the same belief as my sister - that when I found a penny - it was the universe letting me know that everything would be ok. Now, please know I did not look for pennies. I would be walking or riding my bike and happened to look down at the right moment and there would be a penny and sometimes even more.

Haphazardly finding these pennies infused me with the comfort that everything *would* be ok. This feeling was similar to the feeling I have when I walk in nature and connect to her beauty, resilience, strength and her peace.

During September 2019, I was at a point in my life where I was struggling with my decision to give up a well-paying job in pursuit of a more fulfilling and meaningful career. I was feeling financially vulnerable because quite frankly, I was. My small business wasn't doing as well as I hoped, and like others, expenses were escalating at a pace that left me very uncomfortable and sad.

One morning during my visit I decided to go for a walk on the beach by myself and photograph shells and the ocean. I found an interesting shell and decided to use my phone to record its movement as the waves washed over it and tumbled it in the sand. Just when I stopped recording and bent over to resume photographing, what do you think I found slightly buried in the sand? A penny! On that WHOLE ENTIRE SANDY BEACH I PICKED THE SPOT WHERE A PENNY WAS REVEALED to me. I gasped, and in pure delight and gratitude, I looked around, smiled, and silently offered a *Thank You.*

And so...Yes, I too believe...Miracles DO happen. As I stated in this guide...You are a miracle, your body is a miracle and I hope you know deep within your heart - You are not alone AND you have help. On that note, **May you be well and may you wholeheartedly accept that each day is truly a brand new beginning.**

With So Much Love, *Mary*

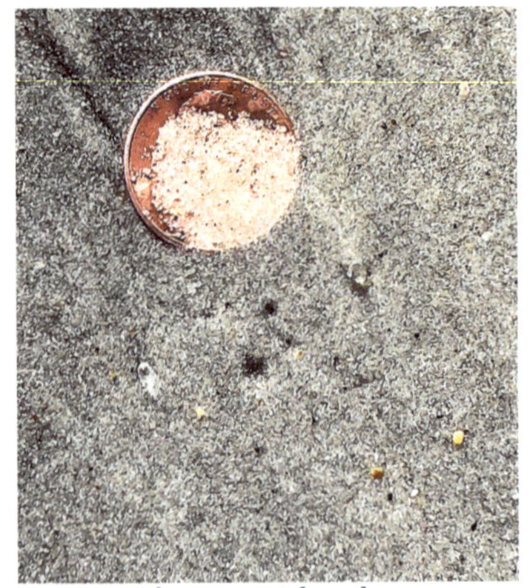

The penny I found

May you
be with
Peace...
for this
too shall
pass.

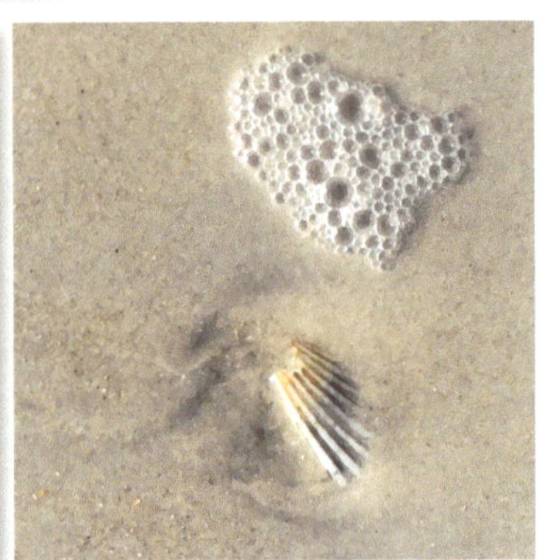

The shell I was recording

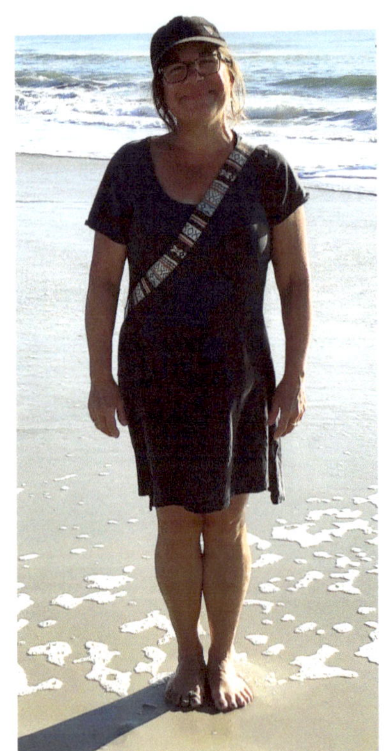

Me, that morning

You are
healing in
so many
ways.

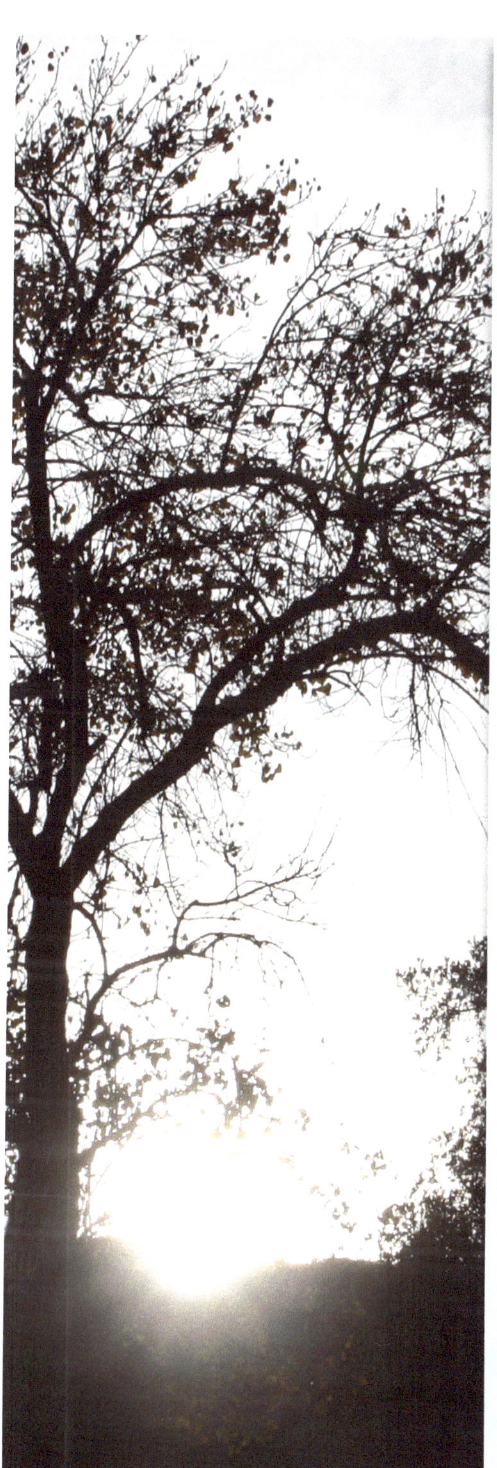

A Brand New Day

What if
One day
You realized
You are FREE
FREE
To listen to your heart
To take care of yourself
To imagine and walk
   toward your possibilities
To express yourself
To summon more of your
   inner strength
To fully believe in you,
and me and us. . .

What if
One day
You woke up
In the very place of
  which you dreamed
And found yourself
  infused with joy and
  peace and so much
  love and appreciation
For the miracle of you
As you are right now
And all you have the
  potential to be
In this beautiful,
  breathtaking, magical,
  challenging,
  magnificent,
  heartbreaking,
  extraordinary
  adventure we call Life
And so...
Let it be.

Until Next Time . . .

I hope this guide has inspired your healing process and that you'll use what you've learned to take even better care of your whole self - body, mind and spirit - throughout your life journey. Be sure to continue your centering breathing, positive thinking and supportive choices. Also, be kind to yourself as the steps in this guide require practice and patience.

For healing and maintaining your overall well-being, mindfulness is one of the best (and scientifically proven) tools available. Anyone can use it as it trancends all ages, races, religions and physical abilities. Mindfulness is simply the practice of being more aware of yourself (thoughts, body, life) in the present moment, *and* invites us to be in relationship with our circumstances in ways that are non-judging, patient, curious, trusting, non-striving, accepting and flexible with what is.

I have imparted the attitudes of mindfulness throughout this guide and encourage you to learn more about them. In addition to a wide selection of online resources (*Helpguide.org* is excellent), I strongly recommend Jon Kabat-Zinn's book, *Full Catastrophe Living*, and also a look at *Mindful Magazine*.

Lastly, I want to emphasize the important principles and energy of love, compassion, gratitude and forgiveness. All are powerful medicine for the heart and soul. Put them in your pockets for your life journey and they will help you get through most anything and accelerate your healing.

I leave you with a little something to contemplate...*With all your experiences so far, what wise advice would you offer to a young child?*
Lastly, ALWAYS remember, **Anything is possible!**